Diabetes

Handy Book

(A Practical Guide)

By Nitin Kulkarni

Contents

Acknowledgments

First and foremost, I would like to thank my Parents and Teachers for educating me and directly helping me in achieving my goals in studies, career, and life.

Next, I am grateful to my wife Aditi, for enduring support throughout the development of this book. Her love and encouragement helped make this book possible

I would also like to thank amazon.com and createspace.com for providing authors like me all the support needed to independently publish our books and market it to the entire world.

I would like to hear from my readers suggestions, or bug reports: nitin.kulkarni79@gmail.com

Nitin Kulkarni

1. Introduction

1.1. Plan of the Book

This book provides you with practical knowledge to control the long term complications of type 2 Diabetes. It covers diagnosis, medicines, life style changes, link between Diabetes and Blood Pressure, link between Diabetes and Heart Disease, link between Diabetes and Urinary Tract Infection (UTI), link between Diabetes and Kidney disease, Ketones, alternative medicines etc.

Diabetes is a chronic disease hence early diagnosis and proper treatment is essential to avoid long term complications. This book provides special emphasis on preventing cardio vascular complications of diabetes.

1.2. What is Diabetes?

Diabetes is when your blood glucose, also called blood sugar, is too high. Blood glucose is the main type of sugar found in your blood and your main source of energy. Glucose comes from the food you eat and is also made in your liver and muscles.

Every cell in our bodies must have a constant source of glucose in order to fuel metabolism. If the cells are unable to get adequate amounts of glucose, they can literally starve to death. As they do, tissues and organs begin to degenerate. A range of 90–120 mg/dL or 90–130 mg/dL before a meal, and less than 140 or 150 (some recommend 180) two hours after a meal is considered normal.

1.3. Types of Diabetes

1.3.1. Type 1 Diabetes

It is also known as Insulin Dependent Diabetes Mellitus (IDDM), and daily insulin injections are required for its treatment. In type 1 diabetes, your body no longer makes insulin or enough insulin due to the damage of the cells that make insulin. In this book we will be focusing mainly on Type 2 Diabetes.

1.3.2. Type 2 Diabetes

It is also known as Non-Insulin Dependent Diabetes Mellitus (NIDDM), and it can be treated with oral medicines, diet, exercise and lifestyle changes. In type 2 diabetes, your body does not produce sufficient insulin and cannot utilize insulin properly due to resistance to insulin.

2. Diagnosis of Diabetes

2.1. Am I suffering from Diabetes?

2.1.1. Fasting Blood Glucose Test

A blood glucose level of 126 mg/dL or higher after an 8 hour fast indicates Diabetes. The test can be sometimes repeated to re-confirm Diabetes.

2.1.2. Oral Glucose Tolerance Test (OGTT)

Please visit your nearby Hospital/Clinic and go through Oral Glucose Tolerance Test. Diagnosis of Diabetes is essential for the physician to prescribe medicines appropriate for you.

Diabetes Symptoms:

- Φ Frequent urination
- Φ Excessive thirst
- Φ Unexplained weight loss
- Φ Extreme hunger
- Φ Sudden vision changes
- Φ Numbness in hands or feet
- Φ Feeling very tired much of the time
- Φ Very dry skin

2.2. Pre Diabetic and Newly Diagnosed Diabetic

Newly diagnosed Diabetic (a person with diabetes) needs time and patience to understand diabetes and learn everything possible to control it properly. Diabetics need to be very cautious with their diet, life style, medicines, drinking and smoking habits.

Tips for newly diagnosed: Include little yogurt/curd in your daily diet.

2.2.1. Managing Post Meal Blood Glucose Level

Blood sugars are highest one hour after eating a meal or snack. Mild exercise after eating can help control the spike in post-meal blood sugars. Glycemic Index (GI) ranks food on how quickly it raises blood sugar levels. Consume only a limited quantity of foods with high Glycemic Index such as Rice, Potatoes, White bread, and most cereals.

Instead of eating 2 big meals, diabetics can plan for eating smaller meals spread throughout the day. It increases digestion and also maintains constant energy and blood glucose level. Maintain a gap of at least 4 hours between (1) Breakfast and Lunch; (2) Evening snack and Dinner.

2.2.2. Self monitor Your Blood Sugar Levels

You can buy a blood glucose monitoring device and measure blood sugar level at home itself. It is very easy to use and safe, and saves your time by helping you to avoid unnecessary visits to the hospital. Self monitoring can reduce vital organ damage by 32% and death incidences by 51% in people with type 2 diabetes.

Steps to check your blood sugar level

Step 1: Prick your finger to get a drop of blood for testing.

Step 2: Apply blood drop on the testing strip of your monitoring device to find the blood glucose level.

2.2.3. Why Yogurt is important?

Diabetic medicines such as Metformin and Insulin can give several side effects, and yogurt can help to nullify these side effects due to its natural properties.

2.2.4. Am I also suffering from High Blood Pressure?

Diabetics usually also suffer from high blood pressure as both these diseases are related to each other.

2.2.5. What is High Blood Pressure?

Blood pressure is the force of blood against artery walls. It is measured in millimeters of mercury (mmHg) and recorded as two numbers i.e. systolic pressure over diastolic pressure. If blood pressure stays elevated over a prolonged time then it is known as High Blood Pressure or Hypertension.

Category	Systolic (mmHg)	Diastolic (mmHg)
Normal	Less than 120	Less than 80
Pre Hypertension	Between 120 to 139	Between 80 to 89
Hypertension	140 or higher	90 or higher

3. Diabetes Medicines

3.1. Which Medicines do I need?

The commonly prescribed medicine is Metformin (generic name). It is the first-line drug of choice for the treatment of type 2 Diabetes and is the only drug that has been conclusively shown to prevent the cardiovascular complications of Diabetes.

Some patients do not adapt to Metformin and starts discontinuing it. More experience/knowledge is required to utilize Metformin effectively. Doctor might also prescribe Insulin in addition to Metformin.

3.2. How to adapt with Metformin?

It depends on how your body is reacting with Metformin.

- Φ Reduce the dosage (usually 500 mg tablets are prescribed but we can also start with 250 mg of Metformin and gradually increase the dosage).
- Φ If you experience side effects with combinations (Metformin+Glimepride) then please discontinue the combination medicine immediately.
- Φ Absorption of Metformin is very slow; hence do not mix Metformin with any other drugs or alcohol.
- Φ Usually diabetics also suffer from High Blood Pressure; hence controlling it is a key to managing Diabetes.

Φ Keep at least once a week completely off from the medicine.

Φ Include little yogurt/curd/probiotic daily.

Φ Perform light exercise like walking, engage in daily household chores, play with your kids etc.

3.3. What precautions do I need to take?

Combining Metformin and Alcohol can be fatal due to the possibility of lactic acidosis, a severe life threatening condition. To be on a safer side always keep some days off from this medicine and split your total dose into multiple lower doses i.e. instead of taking one tablet of 500 mg in the morning split it into two tablets of 250 mg each, one in the morning and another in the afternoon.

3.4. How to adjust with a large dosage?

It is possible that your Doctor might have prescribed a large dosage of the medicine such as 500mg of metformin, twice or thrice daily. It is usually prescribed if your blood sugar is out of control and needed only for short period of time until your blood sugar returns back to normal.

Limiting carbohydrate intake is the best option to bring blood sugar back to the normal range. You need to learn to count the number of calories in various dishes to calculate the total carbohydrates consumed in a day.

3.5. Insulin Shots

Only a doctor can prescribe insulin. You need to learn about Low Blood Sugar (Hypoglycemia) before starting on insulin, always consult your doctor before changing your dosage or discontinuing insulin. Never share insulin needles or insulin pens, even with family.

3.6. Alternative Medicines

Many ancient medicines are available in Ayurveda to control Diabetes such as:

Name of Herb	Benefits
Bitter Melon (Karela)	Strengthens **immunity** and fights Diabetes naturally
Brahmi	Improves Mental Alertness and prevents **Stroke**, particularly beneficial to elderly.
Arjuna Terminalia	Maintains **Heart** health and good for controlling High Blood Pressure (acts like Aspirin).
Ashwagandha	Reduces **Stress**

4. Effect of Diabetes on Human Body

4.1. Diabetes and Human Body

Diabetes is associated with long-term complications that affect almost every part of the body. High blood sugar (Hyperglycemia) can cause damage to many parts of your body such as Kidneys, Eyes, Nerves, Heart, Blood vessels etc. It can also cause Blood Pressure and hardening of the arteries.

4.2. What is Low Blood Sugar?

If your blood glucose levels drop below 70, you have low blood glucose, also called Hypoglycemia. It is caused by taking too much Diabetes medicine, missing or delaying meal, engaging in strenuous activity, drinking alcohol etc. Signs of low glucose are hunger, dizziness, confusion, sweating more, weakness, anxiety etc.

4.3. What is High Blood Sugar?

If your blood glucose levels stay above 180 for more than 1 or 2 hours, you have high blood sugar, also called Hyperglycemia. It is caused by missing medicines, eating too much, have an infection, are stressed etc. Signs of high glucose level are feeling thirsty, feeling tired, headaches, frequent urination, trouble paying attention, blurry vision etc

4.4. Diabetes and Blood Pressure

Usually many diabetics also suffer from High Blood Pressure (BP). Both Diabetes and BP are considered as silent killer and the combined effect can be very dangerous. Controlling both of them can be a challenging job.

Blood Pressure can be controlled by reducing stress and concentrating on one's hobbies. It can also be controlled by taking Aspirin or using alternative medicines given below. Always think positively and learn to relax for at least 30 minutes every day without engaging in any activity/work etc.

· 4.5. Diabetes and Heart Disease

4.5.1. What is Heart Disease?

The term heart disease refers to several types of heart conditions. The most common type is Coronary Artery Disease (CAD), which can cause heart attack. CAD occurs when arteries that supply blood to the heart muscle become narrowed by buildups of fatty deposits called plaque. Other kinds of heart disease may involve the valves in the heart, or the heart may not pump well and cause heart failure. Some people are born with heart disease.

4.5.2. What are the rise factors?

If you smoke, eat an unhealthy diet, and lead a sedentary life, then your risk of having heart disease increases. Having high cholesterol, high blood pressure, or diabetes also can increase your risk for heart disease.

4.5.3. What are the symptoms of heart disease?

You may experience the following symptoms:

Φ Shortness of breath, especially when lying down

Φ Coughing or wheezing, especially when you exercise or lie down

Φ Pain or discomfort in the jaw, arms, shoulder or neck

Φ Weakness, light-headedness, or a cold sweat.

Φ Swelling in feet, ankles and legs

Φ Weight gain from fluid buildup

Φ Confusion or can't think clearly

4.5.4. How is heart disease diagnosed?

Your doctor can perform several tests to diagnose heart disease, including chest X-rays, coronary angiograms, electrocardiograms (ECG or EKG), and exercise stress tests. Ask your doctor about what tests may be right for you.

4.5.5. How to prevent heart disease?

Φ Eat a healthy diet that is low in salt and saturated fat

Φ Exercise regularly

Φ Quit smoking

Φ Avoid drinking spirits such as whisky, rum, brandy, vodka etc.

Φ Red wine in moderation can be beneficial for heart

Φ Control other health conditions such as hypertension, diabetes etc.

4.6. Diabetes and Urinary Tract Infection

Urinary Tract Infection (UTI) can lead to Cancer, Kidney failure etc. and Diabetics are more prone to infection as their natural immunity is affected. Care should be taken to maintain overall hygiene and also include foods that increase immunity such as yogurt/curd, Bitter Melon, Alternative medicines (Herbs) etc.

4.7. Diabetes and Kidney disease

Diabetes is the leading cause of Kidney failure. High levels of blood glucose cause stress on the filtering system in the Kidneys. This damage happens without any symptoms and Kidneys stop working properly. Finally, the Kidneys fail and requires a Kidney transplant or dialysis. We can take following steps to keep our Kidneys healthy:

Φ Keep your blood sugar and Blood Pressure under control

Φ Cut back on salt (less than 1 teaspoon per day)

Φ If you're overweight, take steps to loose weight.

Φ Get the albumin (urine) tests for Kidney disease as often as your health care provider recommends.

4.8. What are Ketones?

You may need to check your blood or urine for ketones if you're sick or if your blood glucose levels are above 240. Your body makes ketones when you burn fat instead of glucose for energy. If you have too many ketones, you are more likely to have a serious condition called ketoacidosis. If not treated, ketoacidosis can cause death.

5. Diabetes and Tests

Test	Frequency	Usage
A1C Test	At least twice a year	Gives average blood glucose level for the past 2 to 3 months.
Blood Lipid Tests	As per the need	Gives LDL, HDL cholesterol and triglycerides details.
Kidney Function Tests	At least once a year	Gives an indication of the kidney damage through urine and blood test
Dilated Eye Exam	At least once a year	Complete eye exam
Dental Exam	At least twice a year	Regular checkup and cleaning

6. Diabetes Control

6.1. What life style changes are needed to control Diabetes?

Cutting down on carbohydrates is the most important point. Light exercise such as walking can be very helpful. If you are suffering from High BP then even regular walking can be fatal hence monitor your Blood Pressure regularly before starting on exercise. About 75% of deaths in diabetics are due to coronary artery disease hence self monitor the blood glucose level and Blood Pressure at home to avoid future complications.

(**Tips**: Never eat too much at any time. A blood sugar above 180 mg/dl over a long period can damage the Kidneys and other vital organs)

6.2. How to deal with stress in Diabetics?

- Φ Relax everyday without performing any task/work for at least 30 minutes.
- Φ Include nutritive rich foods such as fruits, nuts (especially almonds), fiber rich grains, yogurt/curd etc.
- Φ Cultivate a hobby such as painting, playing musical instruments, swimming, playing games, listening to music, reading books etc.
- Φ Perform light exercise such as brisk walking, stretching, yoga etc.

Φ Try to spend more time with kids, family members, friends etc.

Φ Plan for a small travel/holiday with the family or friends.

Φ Always think positively under any circumstances.

Φ Visit religious places such as Churches, Temples, or Mosques etc.

Φ Enroll yourself for a new course.

Φ Improve your skills (communication, presentation, or language skills)

6.3. Can I drink Liquor?

Strictly no. Combining Metformin with alcohol can be fatal. Alcohol directly irritates the stomach and intestines, causing inflammation of the stomach lining and results in abdominal pain, nausea, vomiting and other symptoms.

Many brewery companies spend millions of dollars advertising that drinking is sexy and it will attract more women and all such nonsense just to sell crap and make more money. In reality drinking is the cause of all evil in the society such as accidents, falling sick, assault on women, rape etc.

Drinking effects are three-fold i.e. effect on self (alcoholic), dependents (family members of alcoholic), and unknown from society (physical assault or accidents).

6.4. Can I drink Wine or Beer?

Red wine can actually help to control Diabetes. Generally taking a glass of red wine is not harmful but excessive of red wine can be fatal.

*(**Tips***:If you are planning to drink wine then choose only small amount of medicine i.e. 250 mg of Metformin)*

Beer contains carbohydrate hence it is strictly not recommended for Diabetes.

7. Diabetes and Food

7.1. Which foods diabetics must strictly avoid?

- Φ All soft drinks.
- Φ All types of sweets including chocolates.
- Φ All food products containing white flour like white cookies, cakes, bread, pizza, burger etc.
- Φ All fried products like chips, french fries, donuts etc.
- Φ Sodas (due to high salt)
- Φ Fruit juices (due to added sugar)
- Φ All artificial sweeteners.
- Φ All preserved/frozen foods i.e. prefer to eat only fresh food.

7.2. Which foods diabetics must include?

Food Category	Food Items
Probiotic	Yogurt, Butter Milk, Cheese (in moderation)
Spices	Ginger, Garlic, Cinnamon, Fenugreek Seeds, Cloves, Black Pepper, Cumin, Asafoetida and any other spices. (Caution: Asafoetida is a very strong herb, and only a pinch or one tenth of teaspoon should be enough.)
Cereals	Wheat, Rice, oats, barley, corn, sorghum etc. (All in moderation only)
Vegetables	Tomato, Onion, Cucumber, Carrots, Bitter Melon, Cabbage, Cauliflower, Broccoli, Mustard Greens, Spinach, Fenugreek leaves.
Dry Fruits	Almond, Dry Fig
Fruits	Apple, Orange, Pomegranate, Water Melon

7.3. What is the effect of consuming sugar?

Sugar consumption causes mineral deficiencies especially Zinc, which plays important role in nervous system functioning and wound healing. High sugar increases load on pancreas, liver, and kidneys and damages all these vital organs slowly.

7.4. Why do I feel the urge to consume more sugar?

Sugar consumption is addictive and you are tempted to consume more and more sugar.

7.5. How to stop food craving among Diabetics?

Stay away from junk food with extra salt/sugar in it because spicy foods increase craving and you are tempted to eat more. Eat foods rich in nutrients such as fruits, yogurt, figs, almonds etc. Always prefer food in its natural form instead of processed or refined food that is deprived of vitamins or minerals.

8. What are the contradictions?

Above suggestions are not suitable for persons suffering from Kidney disease, allergic to any of the drugs or persons suffering from type 1 Diabetes.

Additional References

American Diabetes Association

www.diabetes.org

American Association of Diabetes Educators

www.diabeteseducator.org

National Diabetes Education Program

www.ndep.nih.gov

www.yourdiabetesinfo.org

National Diabetes Information Clearinghouse

www.diabetes.niddk.nih.gov

Index